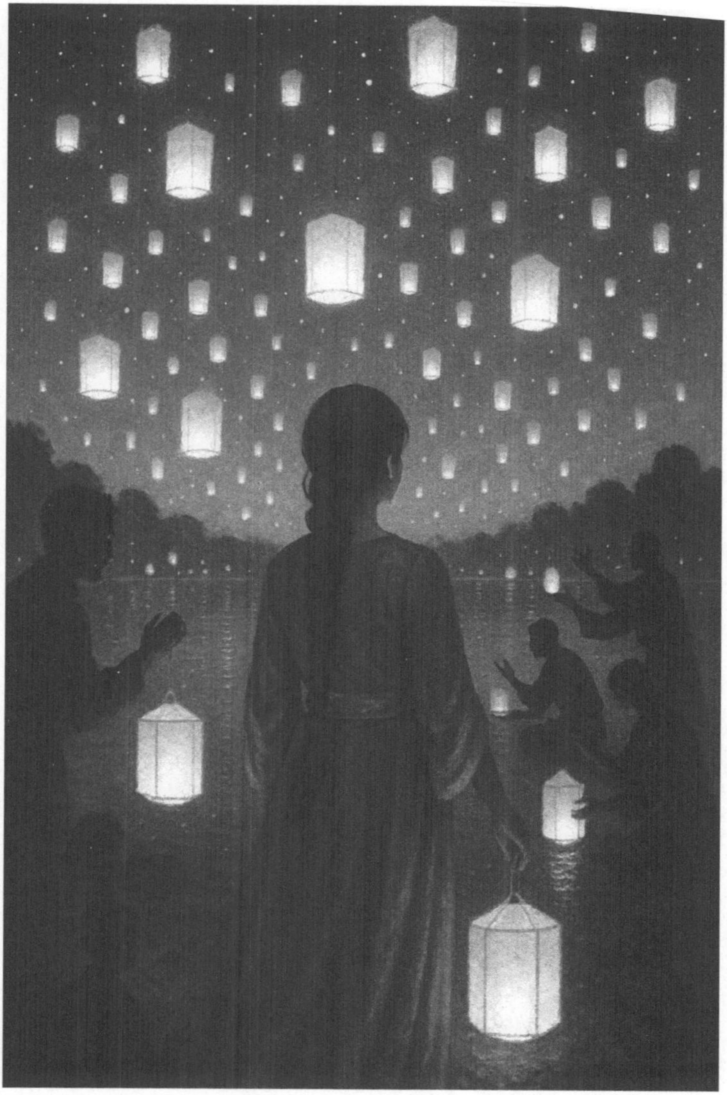

First Published by Ink Gladiators Press®

Translations Of Hope

Editor-in-Chief: Reena Doss

First Edition
ISBN 13: 978-93-49117-94-5

Tree Stones For You - Lantern 5

Credits:

Book Design by Leonie Belle Hawk
Irish & Norwegian Translations: Edited and Proofed
by Justin Adam Wolf and Aelius Arche

Ink Gladiators Press®

Publishing and promoting warriors on life's battlefield

Founded in 2019 | Bangalore, India

www.inkgladiatorspress.com

To my beloved Weaver,

Thank you for the music living in the branches
of green forests, beautiful trees and flower gardens;
this is my joyful thank you to you for adding lyrics
through the unstoppable flow of my oceanic heart

To my future family,

The songs that I am writing are for you;
May you discover the secret threads
I leave in the lines for you to find

To my dear Song Writers—

Here's to us! May we never stop creating music,
adding elements, and voices that suit our genres
May our words bring healing to hearts that need to listen
May our songs touch the ones who feel alone

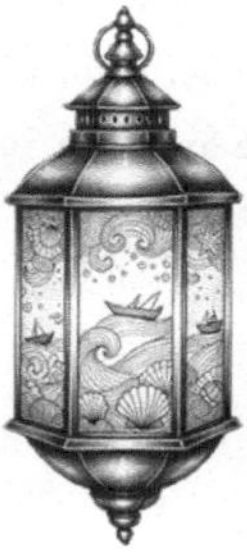

This book is a lantern of

Tree Stones For You

♥

Love Adores
Never-ending Tales:
Eagerly Ready, News Sails

These lyrical works are dedicated to the most surreal trees to have ever existed. Originally written in English, the songs are translated into Irish and Norwegian. The 13 stones, on the other hand, are just decorative added elements meant to reimagine how beautiful each tree would look when painted, framed, and hung in a gallery to admire. Also, Wild Trees Sing is the name of the album that can be found on Suno @reenadoss.

Tree Stones For You

Because Mental Health Matters

I stopped numbering my pages because my story is still being written.

Besides, I do like its symbol a lot—a sleeping 8.

I'll find you in the dark because I'm the girl

who loves to stay *lost* amongst the midnight stars

caught up with moonbeams *in a lantern*

trying to find my way back *home*

LANTERNS

The pleasure of watching light move across the night sky against its deep purples, blues and greys is an incredible sight to behold.

Though I have never seen it in person myself except on TV, reels or videos, I would imagine that it mimics the feeling of a thousand golden suns glimmering brighter than the stars behind them. I would imagine that it would capture the feeling of remembering that we are each important because no matter how small or big we are light travels faster than sound. I would imagine it would make anyone who sees them smile, open their hearts as hope flutters like birdsong near their door, and the taste of something indescribably good wraps them warmly.

Lanterns are necessary because igniting hope is the best cure in support of mental health awareness. Many live in darkness, in a state of feeling disillusioned by those they put their faith in and have forgotten how to see their own hearts through eyes that love, but a lantern is meant for just this purpose—to relight someone's candle with kindness, to hold a hand steadily in their shadows, and to listen gently to the broken pieces in others speaking. Sometimes, the truth is simple.

That delicate point between human nature and the desire to do what is good is where we will meet the Author of Love. Love can only be known from the One who created us and even when people (who follow God) make us feel like He isn't real or there for us, one of the best ways to reconnect with Him directly is to love with all your heart—and to balance it with healthy discernment, boundaries and truth in situations where your broken parts might want to do, feel or say the exact opposite. *E.g.: Jesus Christ*

It is my joy to let go of this lantern—as all lanterns must be—for others to find because I want to share something beautiful that I gained and that is mine to offer: You are deeply loved by Heavenly Hands that have constructed, created and command time, space, and distance.

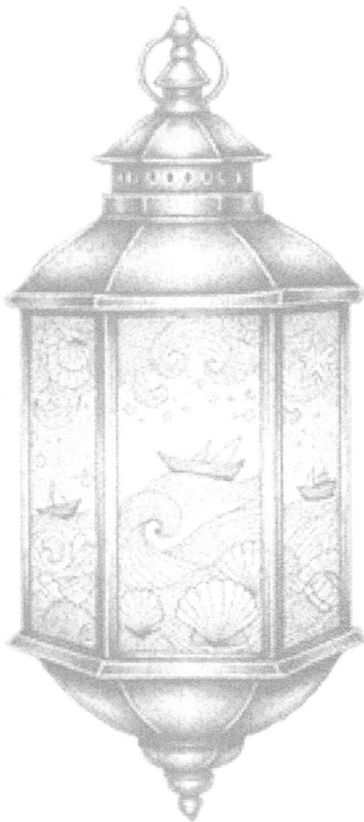

∞

Limestone Painting

Of the Dragon's Blood Tree

Color: Pale, creamy beige, grey, or light brown
Size: 6–8 × 9–12 × 0.5–1 inches | Weight: ~2–3 lbs (0.9–1.4 kg)

Verse:
Bark of the tree, red sap bleeding
Socotra archipelago, resin treasure,
Canopy of the Indian Ocean
Yemen umbrella, timeless without rings
Dragon's blood, Dragon's blood

Sing Verse again

Outro:
Yemen umbrella, timeless without rings
Canopy of the Indian Ocean

Péintéireacht Aolchloiche

Den Chrann Fola an Dragan

Dath: Bán buí éadrom, liath, nó donn éadrom

Méid: 6–8 × 9–12 × 0.5–1 orlach | Meáchan: ~2–3 lb (0.9–1.4 kg)

Verse:

Craiceann an chrainn, sú dearg ag sileadh
Oileandacht Socotra, stór roisín,
Scáthbhrat an Aigéin Indiaigh
Scáth fearthainne an Iemen, síoraí gan fáinní
Fola an dragain, Fola an dragain

Can an véarsa arís

Críoch:

Scáth fearthainne an Iemen, síoraí gan fáinní
Scáthbhrat an Aigéin Indiaigh

Kalksteinsmaleri

Av drageblodtreet

Farge: Blekt, krembeige, grå eller lys brun
Størrelse: 6–8 × 9–12 × 0,5–1 tommer | Vekt: ~2–3 pund (0,9–1,4 kg)

Vers:
Barken på treet, rød saft som blør
Socotra-øygruppen, harpiksens skatt,
Kronetaket over Det indiske hav
Jemen-paraply, tidløs uten ringer
Dragens blod, dragens blod

Syng verset igjen

Outro:
Jemen-paraply, tidløs uten ringer
Kronetaket over Det indiske hav

Slate Stone Painting

Of the Baobabs

Color: Dark gray to black

Size: 7 × 10 × 0.5 inches | Weight: ~2.0 lbs (0.9 kg)

Verse 1:
Dirt road rising
Giant baobabs towering
Breathtaking landscape
Surreal trunks

Chorus:
Your roots are upside down
Reach for the sky,
Reach for the sky

Verse 2:
Madagascar
Spindly branches of legend
Ancient heartbeat
Your roots are upside down

Outro:
Surreal trunks
Reach for the sky (2)
Giant baobabs towering
Reach for the sky (2)

Péintéireacht Cloiche Sclátaí

De na Baobabaigh

Dath: Liath dorcha go dubh
Méid: 7 × 10 × 0.5 orlach | Meáchan: ~2.0 lb (0.9 kg)

Líne 1:
Bóthar cré ag éirí
Baobabanna ollmhóra ag síneadh in airde
Tírdhreach a bhaineann an anáil díot
Gasanna osréalaíocha

Curfá:
Tá do fhréamhacha bun os cionn
Ag síneadh i dtreo na spéire,
Ag síneadh i dtreo na spéire

Líne 2:
Madagascar
Géagáin chaola an fhinscéil
Buille croí ársa
Tá do fhréamhacha bun os cionn

Críoch:
Gasanna osréalaíocha
Ag síneadh i dtreo na spéire (2)
Baobabóga ollmhóra ag síneadh in airde
Ag síneadh i dtreo na spéire (2)

Skifersteinmaleri

Av baobabtrærne

Farge: Mørk grå til svart
Størrelse: 7 × 10 × 0,5 tommer | Vekt: ~2,0 pund (0,9 kg)

Vers 1:
Grusvei stiger
Gigantiske baobabtrær rager høyt
Fantastisk landskap
Surrealistiske stammer

Refreng:
Dine røtter er opp ned
Strekk deg mot himmelen,
Strekk deg mot himmelen

Vers 2:
Madagaskar
Spinkle grener av legender
Gammelt hjerteslag
Dine røtter er opp ned

Outro:
Surrealistiske stammer
Strekk deg mot himmelen (2)
Gigantiske baobabtrær som rager høyt
Strekk deg mot himmelen (2)

Marble Stone Painting

Of the Angel Oak Tree

Color: White, gray, or veined with various hues
Size: 6 × 9 × 0.75 inches | Weight: ~2.5 lbs (1.1 kg)

Verse:
Stories of ghosts,
The people say
John's Island
Giant oaks grow

Chorus:
The soil reveals the past
Sorrows buried
Branches reach to comfort
But angels gather
Angels gather

Outro:
Giant oaks grow
Stories of ghosts
But angels gather
Angels gather

Péintéireacht Cloiche Mármair

den Dharach Aingil

Dath: Bán, liath, nó le féitheanna de dhathanna éagsúla
Méid: 6 × 9 × 0.75 orlach | Meáchan: ~2.5 lb (1.1 kg)

Líne:
Scéalta faoi thaibhsí,
A deir na daoine
Oileán Eoin
Fásann darach mór

Curfá:
Nochtann an chré an t-am atá caite
Brón curtha
Síneann craobhacha le sólás
Ach tagann aingil le chéile
Tagann aingil le chéile

Críoch:
Fásann darach mór
Scéalta faoi thaibhsí
Ach tagann aingil le chéile
Tagann aingil le chéile

Marmorsteinmaleri

Av Angel Oak Tree

Farge: Hvit, grå eller med årer i forskjellige nyanser
Størrelse: 6 × 9 × 0,75 tommer | Vekt: ~2,5 lbs (1,1 kg)

Vers:
Historier om spøkelser,
Folk sier
John's Island
Gigantiske eiketrær vokser

Refreng:
Jorden avslører fortiden
Sorg begravet
Grener strekker seg for å trøste
Men engler samles
Engler samles

Outro:
Gigantiske eiketrær vokser
Historier om spøkelser
Men engler samles
Engler samles

Sandstone Painting

Of the Wych Elm Tree

Color: Reddish-brown, tan, or golden
Size: 8 × 11 × 1 inch | Weight: ~4.0 lbs (1.8 kg)

Verse:
Solitary survivor
From an ancient forest
You are Glenn Affric's pride
Gnarled wisdom
Engraved on your face
Elm Tree
You are centuries old
Last Ent of the tree-folk

Repeat Verse

Péintéireacht Gaineamhchloiche

Den Dair Chaol

Dath: Donnrua, donn éadrom, nó órga

Méid: 8 × 11 × 1 orlach | Meáchan: ~4.0 lb (1.8 kg)

Verse:

Aonaránach marthanach
Ó fhoraois ársa
Is tú bród Ghleann Affric
Eagna ghuairneach
Greanta ar d'aghaidh
Dair
Tá tú na céadta bliain d'aois
An t-Ent deireanach de phobal na gcrann

Aithris an véarsa

Sandsteinsmaleri

Av Wych-almetreet

Farge: Rødbrun, brun eller gylden
Størrelse: 8 × 11 × 1 tomme | Vekt: ~4,0 lbs (1,8 kg)

Vers:
Ensom overlevende
Fra en gammel skog
Du er Glenn Affrics stolthet
Knudret visdom
Inngravert i ansiktet ditt
Almetre
Du er flere hundre år gammel
Den siste av trefolket

Gjenta vers

∞

Granite Stone Painting

Of the Hawthorn Tree

Color: Gray, pink, black, or speckled combinations
Size: 7 × 9 × 1.25 inches | Weight: ~5.0 lbs (2.3 kg)

Verse:
Home to Fairies
Protected and awed
Pink flowers
Red berries
Bees visit

Chorus:
Many roads watch themselves
For you, for you, for you
And Irish homes
Sing, sing, sing
Of your arrival
For you, for you, for you

Outro:
Blossom in May (2)
Blossom bright
For you, for you, for you

Píctiúr Cloiche Gairbhéil

Den Chrann Cuilinn

Dath: Liath, bándearg, dubh, nó meascáin spota
Méid: 7 × 9 × 1.25 orlach | Meáchan: ~5.0 lb (2.3 kg)

Verse:
Teach do na Sióga
Féinchosanta agus faoi gheasa
Bláthanna bándearga
Caora dearga
Tugann beacha cuairt

Chorus:
Bíonn go leor bóithre ag faire orthu féin
Duit, duit, duit
Agus tithe na hÉireann
Can, can, can
Faoi do theacht
Duit, duit, duit

Outro:
Bláthú i mBealtaine (2)
Bláth gile
Duit, duit, duit

Granittmaleri

Av hagtornetreet

Farge: Grå, rosa, svart eller flekkete kombinasjoner
Størrelse: 7 × 9 × 1,25 tommer | Vekt: ~5,0 lbs (2,3 kg)

Vers:
Hjemmet til feene
Beskyttet og ærefryktinngytende
Rosa blomster
Røde bær
Bier besøker

Refreng:
Mange veier passer på seg selv
For deg, for deg, for deg
Og irske hjem
Syng, syng, syng
Om din ankomst
For deg, for deg, for deg

Outro:
Blomstrer i mai (2)
Blomstrer lyst
For deg, for deg, for deg

Soapstone Painting

Of the Rainbow Eucalyptus Tree

Color: Soft gray, greenish, or blue-gray
Size: 5 × 8 × 0.75 inches | Weight: ~1.8 lbs (0.8 kg)

Verse 1:
Bark shedding tree
Why do you hide?
Shy as a rainbow,
You have layers of paint

Verse 2:
Eucalyptus breathes
Into your scented name
Brush strokes of green
Orange, pink, and blue

Chorus:
Purple skies
Found their home in you
Beneath your clothes
Of deep, deep, old brown
Purple skies
Found their home in you

∞

Péintéireacht Chloiche Soip

den Chrann Eoclaipteach an Bhogha Báistí

Dath: Liath bog, glasmhar, nó liathghorm
Méid: 5 × 8 × 0.75 orlach | Meáchan: ~1.8 lb (0.8 kg)

Líne 1:
Crann a scaoileann a bholgán
Cén fáth a bhíonn tú i bhfolach?
Céimneach mar dhath an bhogha báistí,
Tá sraitheanna péinte agat

Líne 2:
An tEucalyptus ag análú
I d'ainm cumhra
Buillí scuab de dhath glas
Oráiste, bándearg, agus gorm

Curfá:
Spéartha corcra
Fuair siad a dteach iatann ionat
Faoi do chuid éadaí
De dhath donn domhain, domhain, sean
Spéartha corcra
Fuair siad a dteach iatann ionat

Täljstenmålning

Av regnbue-eukalyptustreet

Farge: Myk grå, grønnaktig eller blågrå
Størrelse: 5 × 8 × 0,75 tommer | Vekt: ~1,8 pund (0,8 kg)

Vers 1:
Bark som faller av treet
Hvorfor gjemmer du deg?
Sjenert som en regnbue,
Du har lag på lag med maling

Vers 2:
Eukalyptus puster
Inn i ditt duftende navn
Penselstrøk av grønt
Oransje, rosa og blått

Refreng:
Lilla himmel
Fant sitt hjem i deg
Under klærne dine
Av dyp, dyp, gammel brun
Lilla himmel
Fant sitt hjem i deg

∞

Obsidian Stone Painting

Of the Methuselah Tree

Color: Jet black or dark brown, glossy and glass-like
Size: 5 × 7 × 0.5 inches | Weight: ~1.5 lbs (0.7 kg)

Verse 1:
Oh Great Basin Bristlecone
Oldest of your pines
Methuselah, Methuselah

Chorus:
Over four thousand years
Methuselah, Methuselah
Older than the Pyramids of Giza
Methuselah, Methuselah

Verse 2:
California's White Mountains
Protect, listen and hide you
Methuselah, Methuselah

Outro:
Where wind and time sculpt you
Methuselah

Péintéireacht ar Chloch Obsidiáin

De Chrann Mathúsailéim

Dath: Dubh gualach nó donn dorcha, snasta agus cosúil le gloine
Méid: 5 × 7 × 0.5 orlach | Meáchan: ~1.5 lb (0.7 kg)

Líne 1:
Ó a Chrann Britlecone an Mhórghleanna
An seanda de do chuid giúiseanna
A Mhathúsailéim, a Mhathúsailéim

Curfá:
Os cionn ceithre mhíle bliain
Maitéasael, Maitéasael
Níos sine ná Pirimídeacha Giza
Maitéasael, Maitéasael

Verse 2:
Sléibhte Bána California
Cosain, éist agus folúigh thú
Maitéasael, Maitéasael

Outro:
San áit a ndéanann an ghaoth agus an t-am dealbhú ort
Maitéasael

Obsidian Steinmaleri

Av Methuselah-treet

Farge: Kullsvart eller mørkebrun, blank og glassaktig
Størrelse: 5 × 7 × 0,5 tommer | Vekt: ~1,5 lbs (0,7 kg)

Vers 1:
Å, Great Basin Britlecone
Den eldste av dine furutrær
Methuselah, Methuselah

Refreng:
Over fire tusen år
Methuselah, Methuselah
Eldre enn pyramidene i Giza
Methuselah, Methuselah

Vers 2:
Californias hvite fjell
Beskytter, lytter og skjuler deg
Methuselah, Methuselah

Outro:
Der vind og tid former deg
Methuselah

Quartzite Stone Painting

Of the Wollemi Pine Tree

Color: White, gray, pink, or shimmering crystal tones

Size: 8 × 10 × 0.75 inches | Weight: ~4.5 lbs (2.0 kg)

Verse 1:
Chocolate crackles
Living fossil
Relic from the age of dinosaurs
Blue Mountains of Australia
Herald your name in joy

Chorus:
Wollemi Pine, Wollemi Pine
Unusual bark, unique ferns
One of the rarest tree kinds
Wollemi Pine, Wollemi Pine

Repeat Verse and Chorus

Péintéireacht Cloiche Grianchloiche

Den Gharbhán Wollemi

Dath: Bán, liath, bándearg, nó tonnta criostail drithleacha
Méid: 8 × 10 × 0.75 orlach | Meáchan: ~4.5 lb (2.0 kg)

Verse 1:
Ag spréachadh mar sheacláid
Fóisil bheo
Iarsma ó ré na ndineasár
Sléibhte Gorma na hAstráile
Fógraíonn siad d'ainm le lúcháir

Chorus:
Gort Wollemi, Gort Wollemi
Craiceann neamhghnách, raithneach uathúil
Ceann de na cineálacha crann is annamh
Gairbhéad Wollemi, Gairbhéad Wollemi

Athdhéan an Varsa agus an Cór

Kvartsittsteinmaleri

Av Wollemi-furutreet

Farge: Hvit, grå, rosa eller skimrende krystallfarger
Størrelse: 8 × 10 × 0,75 tommer | Vekt: ~4,5 lbs (2,0 kg)

Vers 1:
Sjokolade knaser
Levende fossil
Relikvie fra dinosaurernes tid
Blue Mountains i Australia
Heralder ditt navn med glede

Refreng:
Wollemi-furu, Wollemi-furu
Uvanlig bark, unike bregner
En av de sjeldneste tresortene
Wollemi-furu, Wollemi-furu

Gjenta vers og refreng

Basalt Stone Painting

Of the Montezuma Cypress Tree

Color: Dark gray to deep black
Size: 9 × 12 × 1 inch | Weight: ~6.0 lbs (2.7 kg)

Verse:
Old man of the water
Your waist is jolly and wide
Montezuma Cypress
Your trunk rolls in twists and turns
To make animals come alive

Chorus:
Tree of tule, art is your design
El Árbol del Tule, El Árbol del Tule
Tree of tule, Tree of tule

Repeat Verse
Repeat Chorus Twice

Píctiúr Cloiche Basailt

Den Chrann Cipíníneach Montezuma

Dath: Liath dorcha go dubh domhain
Méid: 9 × 12 × 1 orlach | Meáchan: ~6.0 punt (2.7 kg)

Líne:
A sheanfhear an uisce
Is lánmhaith leathan do choim
A Chraobh-chreasa Mhontezuma
Filleann do chas i gcasadh is i gcuar
Chun ainmhithe a thabhairt chun beochta

Curfá:
A chrann tuile, is ealaín í do dhearadh
El Árbol del Tule, El Árbol del Tule
A chrann tuile, A chrann tuile

Aithris an Líné

Aithris an Churfá faoi Dhó

Basaltsteinmaleri

Av Montezuma-sypressen

Farge: Mørk grå til dyp svart
Størrelse: 9 × 12 × 1 tommer | Vekt: ~6,0 lbs (2,7 kg)

Vers:
Gamle mann av vannet
Din midje er munter og bred
Montezuma-sypress
Din stamme snor seg i svinger og vendinger
For å gi liv til dyrene

Refreng:
Tule-tre, kunst er ditt design
El Árbol del Tule, El Árbol del Tule
Tule-tre, Tule-tre

Gjenta vers

Gjenta refreng to ganger

Dolomite Stone Painting

Of the Banyan Tree

Color: Soft white to light gray
Size: 6 × 10 × 0.75 inches | Weight: ~3.0 lbs (1.4 kg)

Verse 1:
Dear Banyan Tree
Oh little Indian forest
On your own
You expand indefinitely
For people, birds
And animals to shelter

Verse 2:
Dear Banyan Tree
Oh little Indian forest
Aerial roots grow down
From branches
Anchor and create new
Trunks in the soil

Chorus:
Dear Banyan Tree
Oh little Indian forest
Your complexity allows
For infinity

Outro:
Dear Banyan Tree
Oh little Indian forest on your own (2)

Péintéireacht Chloiche Dolamait

den Chrann Bánán

Dath: Bán bog go liath éadrom

Méid: 6 × 10 × 0.75 orlach | Meáchan: ~3.0 lb (1.4 kg)

Véarsa 1:
A Chrann Bánán, a chara
Ó, a choill bheag Indiach
Leat féin
Leathnaíonn tú gan teorainn
Do dhaoine, éin
Agus ainmhithe le foscadh

Véarsa 2:
A Chrann Bhanian ghrá
Ó, a choill bheag Indiach
Fásann fréamhacha aeir síos
Ó na craobhacha
Ag cur faoi agus ag cruthú
Stocanna nua san ithir

Curfá:
A Chrann Bhanian ghrá
Ó, a choill bheag Indiach
Ligeann do chastacht
Don éigríoch

Críoch:
A Chrann Bhanian ghrá
Ó, a choill bheag Indiach leat féin (2)

Dolomittsteinmaleri

Av Banyantreet

Farge: Myk hvit til lys grå

Størrelse: 6 × 10 × 0,75 tommer | Vekt: ~3,0 lbs (1,4 kg)

Vers 1:

Kjære Banyantre
Å, lille indiske skog
På egen hånd
Vokser du uendelig
For mennesker, fugler
Og dyr å søke ly

Vers 2:

Kjære Banyan-tre
Å, lille indiske skog
Luftrøtter vokser ned
Fra grenene
Forankrer og skaper nye
Stammer i jorden

Refreng:

Kjære Banyan-tre
Å, lille indiske skog
Din kompleksitet tillater
Uendelighet

Outro:

Kjære Banyan-tre
Å, lille indiske skog på egen hånd (2)

Schist Stone Painting

Of the Namibian Bottle Tree

Color: Silver-gray, greenish, or brown with reflective flakes
Size: 8 × 9 × 1 inch | Weight: ~3.5 lbs (1.6 kg)

Verse 1:
Silhouette of
Voluptuous temptation
Your water is
Not for consumption

Chorus:
Namibian bottle, Desert wild
Peculiar, strange and otherworldly
Desert wild, Desert wild, Desert wild

Verse 2:
Full of deadly
Poison
Sweet smelling
Pretty flowers

Sing Chorus

Verse 3:
Hunters thank you
For your sap
They coat it
On their arrowheads

Sing Chorus

Péintéireacht ar Chloch Síc

Den Chrann Buidéal Namibiach

Dath: Airgead-liath, glas-liath, nó donn le calóga frithchaiteacha

Méid: 8 × 9 × 1 orlach | Meáchan: ~3.5 punt (1.6 kg)

Verse 1:
Scáthchruth an
Tarraingthe mhór-cháiréil
Ní hé d'uisce
Le hól

Curfá:
Buidéal Namibiach, Fiadha an Fhásaigh
Aisteach, coimhthíoch agus eileolach
Fiadha an Fhásaigh, Fiadha an Fhásaigh, Fiadha an Fhásaigh

Verse 2:
Lán de nimh
mharfach
Bláthanna deasa
a bhfuil boladh milis uathu

Can an Curfá

Verse 3:
Gabha buíochais leat
As do shíológ
Cuireann siad é
Ar bharr a saigheada

Can an Curfá

∞

Skifersteinsmaleri

Av det namibiske flasketreet

Farge: Sølvgrå, grønnaktig eller brun med reflekterende flak
Størrelse: 8 × 9 × 1 tomme | Vekt: ~3,5 lbs (1,6 kg)

Vers 1:
Silhuett av
Fornøyelig fristelse
Vannet ditt er
Ikke til konsum

Refreng:
Namibisk flaske, ørkenens villskap
Særegen, merkelig og utenomjordisk
Ørkenens villskap, ørkenens villskap, ørkenens villskap

Vers 2:
Full av dødelig
Gift
Duftende
Vakre blomster

Syng refreng

Vers 3:
Jegerne takker deg
For saften din
De smører den
På pilspissene sine

Syng refreng

Alabaster Stone Painting

Of the Windswept Trees

Color: White to creamy, sometimes with faint veins
Size: 6 × 8 × 0.5 inches | Weight: ~1.5 lbs (0.7 kg)

Chorus:
Lean, bow and be dramatic
The Roaring Forties
and the Furious Fifties say

Verse:
They bend, shape and warp you
At Slope Point, seen by the land
With speed, strength, and force
They batter the Antarctic Ocean

Sing Chorus

Bridge:
Create a vision
For Nature's racing heart

Sing Chorus

Péintéireacht Cloiche Albastaire

De na Crainn Scairde

Dath: Bán go uachtarach, uaireanta le féitheanna maoile
Méid: 6 × 8 × 0.5 orlach | Meáchan: ~1.5 lb (0.7 kg)

Curfá:
Géill, crom agus bí drámatúil
Deir na Daichead Toirniúla
agus na Caoga Fiáine

Verse:
Lúbann siad thú, múnlaíonn siad thú agus cuaraíonn siad thú
Ag Slope Point, le feiceáil ón talamh
Le luas, neart agus fórsa
Buailíonn siad Aigéan an Antartaigh

Can an Curfá

Droichead:
Cruthaigh fís
Do chroí rásaíochta an Dúlra

Can an Cór

Alabaststeinmaleri

Av vindblåste trær

Farge: Hvit til kremfarget, noen ganger med svake årer

Størrelse: 6 × 8 × 0,5 tommer | Vekt: ~1,5 lbs (0,7 kg)

Kor:
Lene deg, bøy deg og vær dramatisk
De brølende førtiårene
og de rasende femtiårene sier

Vers:
De bøyer, former og forvrenger deg
Ved Slope Point, sett fra land
Med fart, styrke og kraft
Slår de mot Antarktishavet

Syng kor

Bro:
Skap en visjon
For naturens rasende hjerte

Syng refreng

River Stone Painting

Of the Tree Of Life

Color: Naturally varied—gray, brown, tan, or speckled
Size: 3–6 inches | Weight: ~0.3–1.0 lb (0.15–0.45 kg)

Verse 1:
No water source nearby
Yet you survive
Mystical wonder
You dazzle the world

Chorus:
Growing, growing and growing
Oh Mesquite tree on a barren hill
Life emanates from you
In the desert (3)

Verse 2:
Where did you come from?
The people say many things
Tree of Life standing
Still in Bahrain

Sing Chorus

Bridge:
Oh Mesquite tree
In the desert (3)

Péintéireacht Cloiche Abhann

Ar Chrann na Beatha

Dath: Éagsúil go nádúrtha—liath, donn, dath an chraicinn, nó breac
Méid: 3–6 orlach | Meáchan: ~0.3–1.0 lb (0.15–0.45 kg)

Verse 1:
Foinse uisce ar bith in aice láimhe
Ach mar sin féin, maireann tú
Iontas miostéireach
Cuireann tú an domhan faoi dhraíocht

Curfá:
Ag fás, ag fás agus ag fás
Ó, a chrann Mesquite ar chnoc lom
Eascraíonn an bheatha uait
San fhásach (3)

Verse 2:
Céard as a d'eascair tú?
Deir na daoine go leor rudaí
Crann na Beatha ina sheasamh
Go fóill i mBairéin

Can an Curfá

Droichead:
Ó, a chrann Mesquite
San fhásach (3)

Elvesteinmaleri

Av livets tre

Farge: Naturlig variert – grå, brun, beige eller flekkete
Størrelse: 3–6 tommer | Vekt: ~0,3–1,0 lb (0,15–0,45 kg)

Vers 1:
Ingen vannkilde i nærheten
Likevel overlever du
Mystisk underverk
Du blender verden

Korus:
Vokser, vokser og vokser
Å, mesquite-tre på en gold ås
Livet strømmer fra deg
I ørkenen (3)

Vers 2:
Hvor kom du fra?
Folk sier mange ting
Livets tre står
Fortsatt i Bahrain

Syng korus

Bro:
Å, mesquite-tre
I ørkenen (3)

Wild Trees Sing Album

The musical album containing 17 songs can be found at Suno @reenadoss under Creators. Download the app to listen.

♦ Yemen's Umbrella
Tribute to Yemen's Dragon's Blood Tree

♦ Upside Down Roots – (Solo & Chorus Edition)
Tribute to the Avenue of the Baobabs in Madagascar

♦ Ghosts and Angels
Tribute to the Angel Oak Tree in South Carolina

♦ Last Ent
Tribute to the Wych Elm Tree in the Scottish Highlands

♦ Blossom In May
Tribute to the Hawthorn Tree in Ireland

♦ Purple Skies
Tribute to the Rain Eucalyptus Tree found in tropical rainforests

♦ Methuselah
Tribute to a 4,857-year-old Great Basin Bristlecone Pine Tree in California

♦ Wollemi Pine – (Solo & Chorus Edition)
Tribute to the Wollemi Pine Tree in Australia

♦ Old Man Of The Water
Tribute to El Árbol del Tule (Tree Of Tule) in Mexico

♦ Little Indian Forest
Tribute to the Banyan Tree in India

♦ Desert Wild
Tribute to the Namibian Bottle Tree

♦ Roaring Forties And Furious Fifties – (Solo & Chorus Edition)
Tribute to the Windswept Trees at Slope Point

♦ Tree Of Life – (Solo & Chorus Edition)
Tribute to the Mesquite Tree Of Life in Bahrain

∞

Tree Stones For You

Space For You

Reena Doss

Space For You

∞

Tree Stones For You

Space For You

Reena Doss

Acknowledgements

I am grateful

Writing lyrics has been nothing but pure joy from the moment I started taking this voice seriously. At first, I wasn't even aware I was doing it, until one day in early 2018, I found myself singing the words as I was penning them down. That was when it struck me that I could actually be a lyricist. It made me reflect on my childhood and how I used to make up my own words whenever I had a melody in my head. Sometimes, it would happen while I was talking casually to the Weaver, Mother Mary, or the Holy Spirit, or while hearing people I love—my parents, uncles, aunts, and cousins—sing.

In 2022, I published my first collection of lyrics in my second book, *Swallowing The Moon*, never imagining that in just a few years, AI would make it possible for me to create music for my own lyrics. This year, I published my first musical booklet along with its album on Suno, which brought me immense joy and was deeply therapeutic as I found freedom in adding both voice and sound to my words.

This book holds secret lyrical lines for my future husband—the love of my life and best friend forever and ever—according to the Weaver's will, of course. I thank my Heavenly Father for this beautiful gift of lyric writing, imagination, and for the talented artists, performers, and influencers on Instagram who share so many posts about trees, music, and their deep love for nature, echoing my own joy in His creation. I also thank Ink Gladiators Press' team—Leonie Belle Hawk, Justin Adam Wolf, and Aelius Arche—for assisting me with book design, layout, formatting, editing, and proofing.

May the quill of hope find you in the dark,

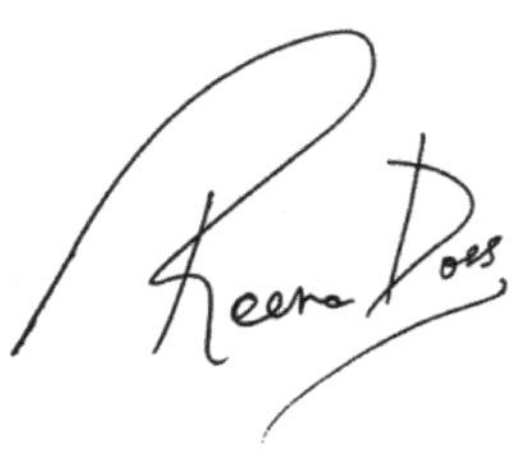

Reena Doss

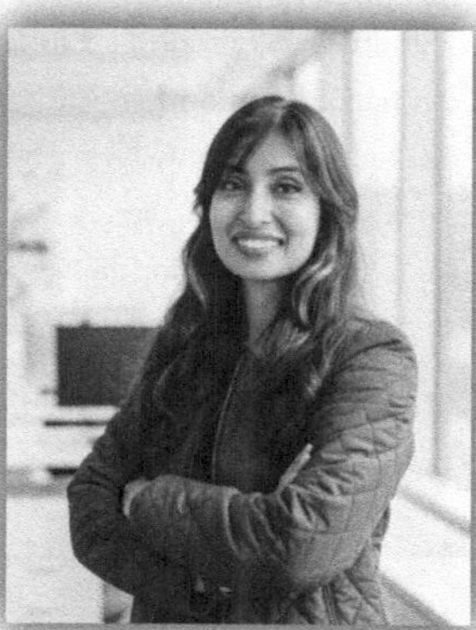

I'll find you in the dark...

Born in Calcutta with roots drawn from Chennai and Pondicherry, Reena Doss has lived most of her life in the south of India—Bangalore. Though she prefers traveling to far-off places inside her head, she sometimes ventures into the world that others call real.

Reena Doss considers writing to be her first voice of expression, followed closely by art, and creativity. Through the encouraging platform provided by the Instagram community, she reclaimed her lost voices, evolved a few others and discovered new ones along the way.

This has redeemed her trust that consistent Hope, Faith and Love in what is true ignites what is impossible to occur. Her adoration for her beloved Weaver, the Celestial Sky, Nature and her fellow Earthians has given her immeasurable courage to endure every season with a resilience born from battles overcome.

You can try and catch her but it may not always be possible as she is generally off on adventures flying on phoenix wings, swimming into the deep with mermaids and chasing fiery dragons down for stories.

To those who remain true to themselves,
to those who create magic wherever they go,
and for those who sit beside the hurt
when everyone else leaves,
Art will always immortalize you.

Please scan the QR code to follow her on
Instagram @reenadossauthor
www.reenadoss.com

This little book is called a *Lantern* because love is light in disguise. It can only be found when you are buried in the dark, when the seeds die, and you choose to bravely grow and become worthy of your given name—a polished gem, a diamond that cannot help but shine. Lanterns are meant for those who need hope while they are being:

- ♥ Condemned unjustly by those who see a version they want
- ♥ Gossiped about when they are not present to defend themselves
- ♥ Taken advantage of when they were beaten down by life, by those who should have stood by them
- ♥ Judged, neglected, and persecuted while they are struggling
- ♥ Abandoned by those who willingly chose to see them as toxic because it suited their narrative
- ♥ Manipulated by those who bore false witness against them to take what wasn't theirs
- ♥ Gaslit, broken, and their truth erased while they were at their most vulnerable
- ♥ Hated, harassed, and purposefully pressured into giving up on who they are because of others' jealousy
- ♥ Trying to process trauma to speak in a language that isn't being heard
- ♥ Eagerly isolated by loved ones on the advice of others who can't understand them any more
- ♥ Neglected by those whose promises dimmed when things got difficult
- ♥ Treated as outcasts by those who expect their will to be done
- ♥ Mocked for what they do just because it is different and does not fit into any box

Promoting hope and unwrapping the stigma of mental health

For any inquiries, please email us at contact@inkgladiatorspress.com.

Please scan the QR Code below if you would like to follow us

on Instagram @inkgladiatorspress.

Ink Gladiators Press®

Publishing and promoting warriors on life's battlefield

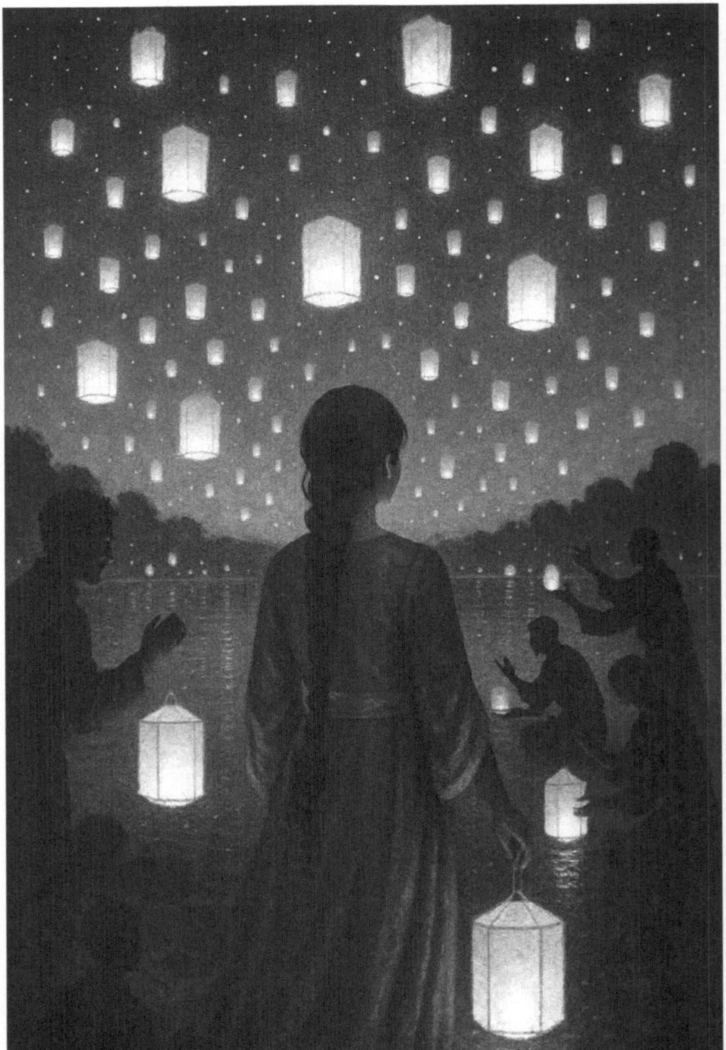

9 789349 117945

Printed at Repro India Ltd.